NATURAL BREAST EXPANSION WITHIN 15 DAYS WITHOUT SURGERY.

ANGELA SPEARS.

TABLE OF CONTENTS

INTRODUCTION

Naturally, woman's body is what defines her beauty, and how she looks at herself is the most important thing to her. That is why before a lady steps out of her house, she must look at the mirror twice or more to make necessary adjustment. The women's appearance and beauty are greatly influenced by their breasts.

The most important thing is to have the right size. You are blessed if you have the ideal breast size. Some women have larger breasts, while others are working towards having larger breasts.

Finding the ideal size and shape presents a challenge. A woman's self-confidence is directly related to her appearance.

She feels low esteemed and unsatisfied with her appearance when she does not have the size she wants.

You can agree with me that large numbers of men prefers women with firmer, supple, fuller and good size of breasts than ‘tangerine’ or smaller boobs sizes.

Research has shown that, ladies with smaller breasts or boobs are being ridiculed by loved ones daily and this has made them to look out for solutions. That is why expansion or enlargement of breast in a natural way without undergoing surgery is necessary.

Breast is the most essential part of the body that attracts men to women. Do not forget that Ladies with good boobs are always complimented by their men.

Naturally, dudes will love to suck and play with them for fun.

Though some women have given up hope and accepted the fact that the "myth" that there is nothing they can do to increase their breast sizes is just a lie.

The simple and proven methods in this book are sure ways to increase your breast size within 15 days and boost your confidence without undergoing surgery.

SIMPLE STEPS TO BREAST ENLARGEMENT.

The size of your breasts is primarily what defines your figure, that is why you have to increase your breast size in a way that will make your body appear more subtle. You need to work hard to reduce sagging, make them stand out and look perfect.

The following steps are important:-

1. The new way to increase your bust size is with silicone cutlets, also known as chicken cutlets or silicone bra cutlets. If you want to instantly increase the size of your breast, it is a good idea to buy these cutlets. You only need to place them on both breasts beneath your bra. Cutlets

contribute to the illusion that your breasts are larger than their actual size in the cup.

2. Select the appropriate bra size: - It is crucial to select the appropriate bra size. A mistake for your breasts is to wear a bra that is either larger or smaller than your size. Your breasts will appear smaller than they are when you wear a bra that is larger than your normal size.

If you want to avoid making this mistake, take a measurement of your bust size and determine your cup size. Therefore, when shopping for a bra, ensure that you select a size that is both appropriate for you and not too big for you.

3. Wear clothes with striking patterns and colors. Don't let your jeans or anything else at the bottom of your outfit look as dark as your tops. Make your top your focal point. Choose tops with bold patterns and colors and bright colors. Try to wear a top with two colors on it. Check to see that the color below your breasts is more striking than the color above. It makes your breasts appear more popped out and perked up. Additionally, horizontally striped tops aid in creating the illusion of larger breasts. Therefore, when you go shopping, keep these considerations in mind and select your top accordingly.

4. Higher neckline women with smaller bust sizes should opt for tops with a

higher neckline. Since wearing clothes with a lower neckline reveals what you are trying to conceal, they are designed for people with larger bust sizes and not smaller bust sizes.

5. Do-It-Yourself halter neck bra creating a do-it-yourself halter neck bra is the simplest way to make your breasts appear larger. You just need to replace the worn-out bra. Remove the straps from the bra's backside. The front steps shouldn't be cut.

6. You can now make it a halter neck bra by tying the straps around your neck. The appearance of a larger cup size is created by halter-neck bras. It

accentuates your cleavage by lifting the breasts.

7. The traditional method of naturally and significantly increasing bust size is breast massage. Massage not only makes the breasts bigger, but it also softens them and gives them the perfect shapes. There are numerous methods for massage. Breast massage is one such method.

Place your palms on your breast to begin. Then, start circularly rubbing your breasts. Your left hand should move in the opposite direction of your right hand. Press your breasts down while moving inward. Instead of just rubbing your hands against them, your breasts should move and rotate on their own. To achieve the desired result, practice this rotation at least 10 times.

Research has that massaging your breast increases blood flow and stimulate collagen production, which may give you a little lift by tightening your muscles and encouraging the growth of new tissue.

To give your breasts a massage:

- Begin by cupping one hand on the opposite breast's top.

- Gently squeeze the area while pumping in a rhythmic motion.

- Slowly move your hand down your breast's top.

• Using the same pumping motion, work your hand around the inside, underside, and outside of your breast.

• Use gentle circles with your fingertip to switch between squeezing and pumping.

8. A padded or push-up bra is probably the simplest way to instantly make your breasts appear larger and fuller. Choose a padded or push-up bra size that is neither too small nor too big. You do not need to add any stuffing; this bra is sufficient to achieve the goal of making your breast appear larger.

9. The most recent trend is the cleavage facial. The cleavage facial is a type when you want to increase your boobs size, you do not always need cutlets or bronzer.

You only need to take care of the breast skin. The skin around the breasts becomes more supple thanks to this unique cleavage. This makes it smoother and more appealing, which makes it even more appealing.

10. Using contouring makeup can give the appearance of a larger breast. One of these is contouring. The only thing left to do is select the appropriate bronzer shade for contouring. To make it appear to be deeper, apply it to your cleavage. Your breasts appear heavier when you have deeper cleavage.

11. Wearing tops with a detailed neckline are your best option. The tops with a few twists and pleats, beads, jewels, and

lace. Your breast will appear appropriate thanks to these details, which will assist in deflecting attention.

12. Socks are the solution when you suddenly plan a night out and don't have a push-up or padded bra to match your dress, stuffing your bra is a good idea. You only require socks, and any socks, regardless of size, will suffice. Simply fold the socks in half or fold them so that they are the size of your hands. Now stuff it into your breasts' sides. With little effort, stuffing socks gives the impression of deeper cleavage.

13. Reduce your waistline: - not working out and exercising, because working out will definitely help you lose weight, but

there are other ways to do it. Wear a high-waist clothes and you can add a belt to your dress which will make it more fitted and appropriate. To make your waist appear slimmer, you can also wear specialized girdles and straps that are available in the market.

Body shapers are another option that can improve your figure and make you look better. This will make you look elegance, giving the impression that your breasts are bigger, this is the secret of most celebrities.

14. Double bra! Wearing two bras simultaneously may sound bizarre and insane. You might wonder whether or not this will actually make the breast appear

larger. It will undoubtedly help you appear to have larger breasts. The second bra you have piled on top of your first bra raises your breast even more than the first bra did.

15. Choose a bra with side boning, you should choose a bra with side boning. Boning aids in breast elevation. It puts the breasts in the middle of the chest, making them look their best.

16. Another way to make your breasts stand out and appear larger on their own is to pin them in your bra. Additionally, this method aids in achieving a deep cleavage. Paper clips or safety pins are both options for pinning. All that is required of you is to tie the back straps

together. The paper clip is the only option if you don't want to see holes in your favorite bra. Simply determine the optimal pin position for your bra—one that is neither too high nor too low.

17. Better posture has a significant impact on your breast size. Avoid slouching and sit with your spine straight. A woman who hunches frequently typically gives the impression that her breasts are larger than they actually are. Do not fold your arms across your breast; instead, raise your shoulders and keep your arms by your side.

18. Accessories:- Make use of necklaces, nickels, chains, and other accessories. Your breasts will stand out more when

you wear a pendant on a long chain. A shorter necklace with a larger pendant will also work to give the impression of a larger figure.

19. Avoid wearing a bra for more than four months because its ability to lift your breasts does not last beyond that point. Stand in front of the mirror while wearing your bra. Now examine whether or not your bra is functioning appropriately. If not, you need to get a new one. Because of these kinds of bras, your breasts look smaller than they really are because they sag.

20. Supplement: - Thanks to advances in science, you can now simply take medicines to help your breasts grow in

size with good shapes without undergoing surgery. There are numerous herbal medicines on the market that are the best because they are made of natural, risk-free herbs.

One of these herbal capsules does not have any side effects, making them more dependable and trustworthy.

The breasts become firmer and larger as a result of this medication. It provides a deeper cleavage and lifts the breasts. It not only makes the breasts bigger, but it also makes the skin around them look better and makes them round, healthy, and firm.

21. Wear a shirt that is a little tighter:-

One more simple way to make your

breasts look bigger is to wear a top that is one size smaller than you are. Wear a dress that is small for you, a shirt that no longer fits you. Wearing clothing that is small does not mean that it is difficult for your body to fit into. You can also make your shirt tighter by pining it from the back and covering it with a jacket to hide the tightening techniques.

22. Another way to improve breast circulation is with hydrotherapy. According to a study, hydrotherapy promotes breast firmness by increasing overall blood flow and stimulating nerves.

It is necessary to at least once a day:

• After taking a shower, turn off the water.

• Give your breasts a quick rinse with warm water.

• Rinse your breasts once more with cool water for 30 seconds to have the desired result.

7 BEST ACTIVITIES TO HAVE BIGGER BREAST.

Free weight chest press focuses on the pectorals as well as your shoulders, and rear arm muscles. In the event that you don't have a bunch of hand weights, you can likewise utilize water bottles. Also chest activities can affect bosom size? increment in size, strength, perseverance, and tone of your leg or arm muscles, it can modify your chest muscles.

You can do the activities using the following stages.

1. Snatch a bunch of free weights and hold one in each hand. Pick a weight that

you can press something like multiple times.

2. Lie with your knees twisted, feet level on the floor and somewhat separated.

3. Keep your head on the floor or seat, start the press by broadening your arms over your chest, palms confronting away from your face drawing your paunch button into your spine.

5. Gradually twist the two elbows until they are lined up with the ground.

6. Stop. Then, at that point, rehash, squeezing the weight above until the two arms are completely broadened.

7. Do 2 to 4 arrangements of 5 to 6 redundancies.

At this point, when you attempt this exercise you will feel precisely good. Alternately, start with wall pushups.

1. Start in a high plank on the floor with your wrists stacked under your shoulders.

2. Brace your middle and press the ground away with your palms. Move your shoulder blades down your back and away from your neck.

3. After that, bend your elbows along your entire body to lower yourself toward the floor.

4. Your chest should be about one to two inches above the floor when you lower down. Press your body back to the

starting position after a brief pause and exhalation.

FOODS THAT HELPS TO ENLARGE BREAST SIZES.

Eat a healthy diet, Studies have shown that eating a diet high in nutrients will help you keep your breast tissue healthy and strong.

Use Maca Root: - for thousands of years, maca has been a staple in South American cuisine for centuries and has become a popular natural nutritional supplement. With the first published descriptions of maca roots dating back to 1553, this has been used by humans for centuries.

Maca is known for its tonic properties, so it helps relieve stress factors in the body while maintaining homeostasis. It is also known for its traditional benefits, and limited research shows that it increases and supports stamina and mood.

Simply remove the oil and apply this oil on your chest. Massage gently. Keep this remedy for a few days. This is a natural strategy for red clover breast enlargement; this natural herb is very beneficial. Full breast development is possible with phyto- estrogens and ginseng.

- SOY PRODUCTS

It is commendable to include soy products in the daily diet. Soybeans are rich in phyto-estrogens. This chemical compound provides natural estrogen to the body. Do you need this chemical?

Yes, because estrogen is the hormone that makes breasts plump when a woman has her period.

- FRUITS AND VEGETABLES

Not everyone who has a larger bust is fat. You still need fruits and vegetables to keep your diet balanced. Fortunately, there are a few things that can help with cup size.

Focus on plants that are rich in phyto-estrogens. Estrogen is a hormone in the female body which controls the breast size in the female body. Thus, by taking estrogen rich foods regularly, your breasts will start to grow.

There are a few that are not as concentrated as soy products, but have lower levels of the chemical. Edibles like carrots, cherries, yams etc.

- ❖ SPICES

Finally, add fresh herbs to the plate. Some herbs contain phyto-estrogens. Hence, it is advisable to eat them whenever possible. Certain herbs can also help restore healthy breast tissue.

In summary, eating the following boost your breasts expansion speedily: -

- More nuts, fish, soybeans, pumpkin seeds, and avocados to get more omega-3 fatty acids.

- More eggs and monounsaturated fats to help breast tissue grow.

• More foods high in antioxidants like cabbage, watermelon, and whole grains to keep tissue healthy.

Maintain a healthy weight.

A slimmer waist will make your bust look bigger because your breasts will be closer to your waist.

Finally, to maintain a healthy weight, consume a diet rich in fruits and vegetables and exercise for 30 minutes each day, at least four days per week.

PROCEDURES FOR BREAST EXPANSION

Exercises that focus on the shoulders, back, and chest can help tone the muscles below the chest.

HAND CIRCLES

Hand circles are exactly the same shape. Your weights, boxes or small water bottles to add extra resistance to this exercise.

WALL PRESS

The wall press is a modified version of the pushup you know. Support yourself with a wall or other vertical source. First, face a wall and place your palms close to chest level. Slowly lower yourself while keeping your back straight until your front almost touches your face. Raise your arms and return to the starting position. Repeat the procedure 5-10 times.

ARM PRESS

A handshake is similar to a hand circle. But instead of drawing a circle next to your body, stretch your arms forward. For more advanced moves, try hand weights or use a resistance band. Starting in a seated or standing position, extend your arms forward and bring your palms together. Extend your arms and pull back until your back is arched. Stretch your hands and repeat the movement for just a minute.

HORIZONTAL CHEST PRESS

Like the arm press, this exercise involves pulling the arms towards the front of the body. This is another exercise that works the chest muscles.

• Start with your arms in front of you first with your arms bent at a 90-degree angle Keep your arms folded, open as much as possible Bring your arms together Repeat the movement every minute

PRAYER POSITION

The prayer pose is another exercise that works the chest muscles. It's like the horizontal chest press, except instead of pulling them together; you pull them towards your chest. Stretch your arms out in front of your body, keeping them at shoulder height press your palms together for 30 seconds then join your palms together and bend your elbows at a 90 degree angle Bring your arms to your chest in prayer position and hold 10 seconds blocked. Release Repeat this movement 15 times. All the mentioned exercises can be performed without additional equipment or even without going to the gym. But if you want an extra challenge, you can use resistance bands or small arm weights.

HOW TO CORRECT POOR POSTURE.

Maintaining good posture not only helps to keep your body in proper alignment, but it can also give the impression of lift to your bust.

Maintaining awareness of how you are holding your body is essential to correcting poor posture. It won't change right away, but with time and practice, you might end up with good posture without even realizing it.

STAND POSITIVELY

Observe your posture. If you sit up straight, you can instantly lift your bust. When you are standing, sitting, or lying down, your posture is the position in which you hold your body. When you have good posture, your body is perfectly aligned to support against gravity. You may not be conscious of your posture, but years of poor posture may have brought it to your attention.

Pose your body right and give the impression of larger, more buoyant breasts.

STANDING POSITION

- Keep your weight evenly distributed.
- Stand on your heels.
- Keep your knees slightly bent and your feet shoulder-width apart.
- Tuck your tummy in .

- Keep your head level whenever possible with your earlobes in line with your shoulders.

To naturally grow bigger boobs, strengthen the muscles under your bust by exercising, this make it look like there is more lift.

Alternately, you might modify your diet and include more healthy oils and fats. You can't choose where you gain weight, though. Therefore, if you choose this route, you can also gain additional inches on other areas of your body.

Last but not least, you can adjust your posture. The natural fullness of the breasts may be obscured by hunched shoulders. These suggestions may be all you need to naturally increase your breast size when used in conjunction with exercise or a particular diet.

It is essential to keep in mind that topical estrogen hormone replacement therapy and over-the-counter breast enlargement creams are not the same thing. Breast enlargement can be aided by prescription estrogen hormone replacement therapy.

You can incorporate chest-specific exercises into your overall fitness routine to enhance pectoral strength, function, and tone.

Increasing the strength and size of your pectoral muscles will significantly increase your breast size.

Keep in mind that you don't have to undergo surgery to get beautiful breasts. Exercise helps you fight gravity and aesthetic hacks. It also helps you feel more confident, including in your breasts.

CONCLUSIONS

Ladies! Use no technique that hurts your breast or causes discomfort even though you want to look flawless in your favorite dress. Flaunts your natural endowment after all, you are the only thing greater than yourself. So ladies that have a sweetheart allowed him to play with those boobs, contact and suck them, then you will see the distinction sooner or later.

Get a bra that fits right. According to research, 35% of women wear the wrong size of bra. A bra that fits right gives you the most support, lifting your breasts and keeping your shape.

To determine your actual bra size, you should get fitted by a professional at least

Make sure to discuss your breast shape with your specialist. The kind of bra you buy will depend on how round, asymmetrical, or saggy your breasts are.

Invest in a push-up bra because they are suitable for all types of breasts, a push-up bra is a wardrobe essential. You will get support and lift from a push-up, making your breasts appear fuller and enhancing your cleavage.

More so, taking supplements/ medications, can be optional in order to avoid side effects, is also beneficial.

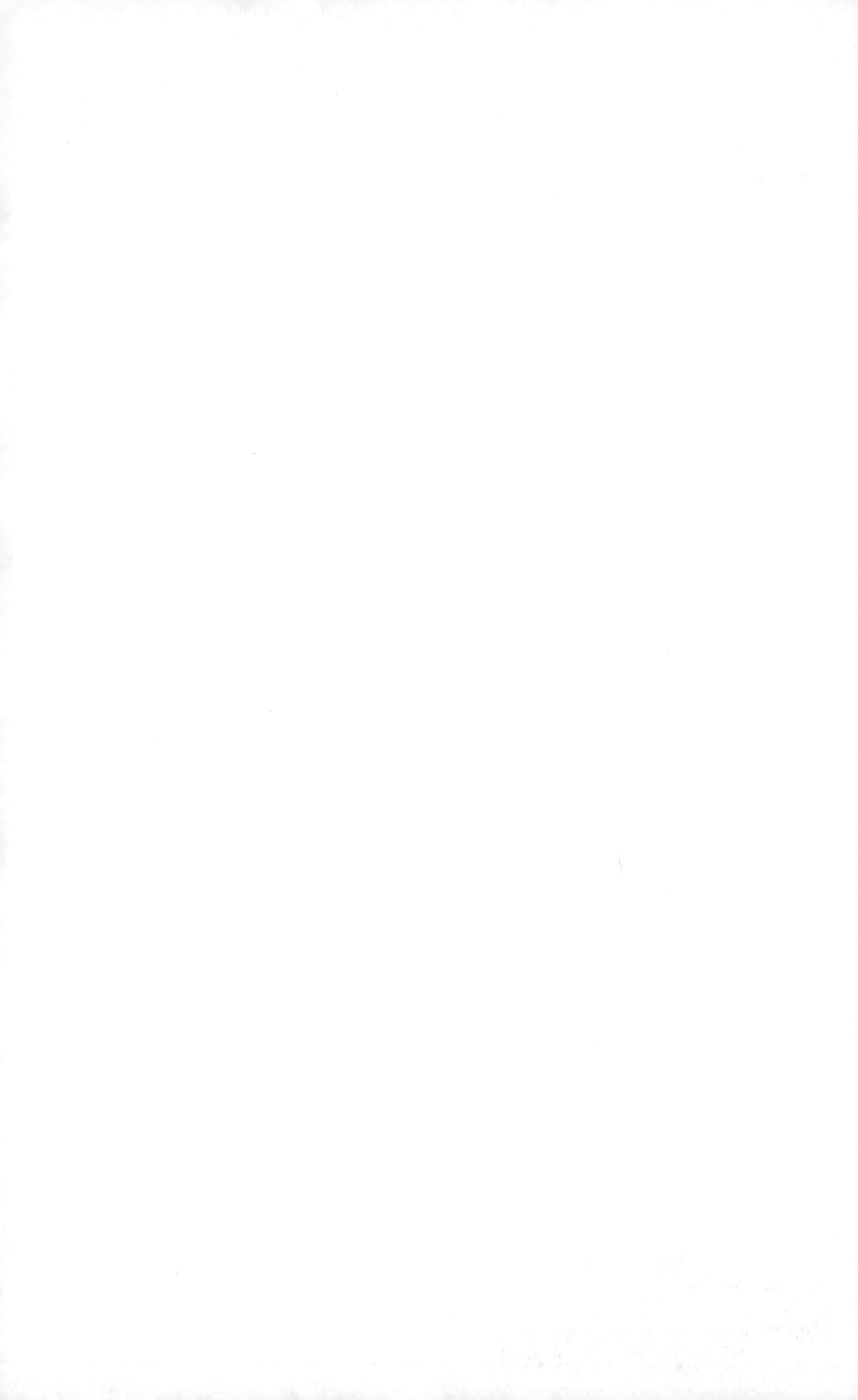

www.ingramcontent.com/pod-product-compliance
Lightning Source LLC
LaVergne TN
LVHW020528160826
845677LV00015B/3959
* 9 7 9 8 3 6 2 8 9 7 0 7 9 *